HERBS—INSTRUMENTS OF SELF HEALTH CARE

Simpler and cheaper than prescription drugs and innocent of troublesome side effects, herbs can perform first aid treatment as well as any other form of remedy, if the basic, necessary information is right at hand. That is efficiently provided in this Health Guide by John Heinerman, herbal expert, who has gathered his facts from the best of the world's herbalists and from his own dedicated research. His recommendations cover minor and major emergencies from cuts to fractures, insect to snake bites, poison ivy to heat stroke or frostbite to gangrene—and almost any other first-aid situation needing help until specialized help arrives.

ABOUT THE AUTHOR AND EDITORS

John Heinerman is a medical anthropologist whose travels in search of information for articles, books and lectures have taken him to China, Russia, India and into almost every corner of the world. He is the author of ten books dealing with herbs and their nutritional and medical applications, and lectures frequently to students and before a variety of lay and professional meetings. Mr. Heinerman is the author of *The Science of Herbal Medicine, The Treatment of Cancer with Herbs* and another Health Guide, *Aloe Vera, Jojoba and Yucca*. His newest book, the first to be written on the subject, is *The Complete Book of Spices: Their Medical, Nutritional and Culinary Uses*.

Richard A. Passwater, Ph.D., is one of the most called-upon authorities for information relating to preventive health care. A noted biochemist, he is credited with popularizing the term "supernutrition" largely as a result of having written two bestsellers on the subject—*Supernutrition: Megavitamin Revolution* and *Supernutrition for Healthy Hearts*. His other books include *Easy No-Flab Diet, Cancer and Its Nutritional Therapies* and *Selenium as Food & Medicine*. He has just completed a new book, *Trace Elements, Hair Analysis and Nutrition* with Elmer M. Cranton, M.D.

Earl Mindell, R.Ph., Ph.D., combines the expertise and working experience of a pharmacist with extensive knowledge in most of the nutrition areas. His book *Earl Mindell's Vitamin Bible* is now a million-copy bestseller; and his more recent *Vitamin Bible for Your Kids* may very well duplicate his first *Bible's* publishing history. Dr. Mindell's popular *Quick & Easy Guide to Better Health* was published by Keats Publishing.

FIRST AID WITH HERBS
TRIED AND TRUE HEALTH CARE IN EMERGENCIES AND MINOR ILLNESSES
by John Heinerman

Keats Publishing, Inc.   New Canaan, Connecticut

First Aid with Herbs is not intended as medical advice. Its intention is solely informational and educational. Please consult a medical or health professional should the need for one be warranted.

FIRST AID WITH HERBS

Copyright © 1983 by Keats Publishing, Inc.

All Rights Reserved

No part of this book may be copied or reproduced in any form without the written consent of the publisher.

ISBN: 0-87983-304-1

Printed in the United States of America

Good Health Guides are published by Keats Publishing, Inc.
27 Pine Street (Box 876)
New Canaan, CT 06840

Contents

	Page
Basic First Aid	1
Cuts, abrasions, minor wounds	2
Diarrhea	2
Frostbite	3
Insect bites and stings, nonpoisonous	3
Nausea and dizziness	4
Parasites	4
Rash and itching	5
Sunburn	5
Emergency Medicine	6
Bites and stings, poisonous (insects, snakes, scorpions, spiders, rabid animals, etc.)	6
Blindness, temporary (caused by chemicals or acids)	9
Burns (first, second and third degree)	10
Choking	13
Fevers (malaria, typhoid, spotted, etc.)	13
Fractures and sprains	15
Heat stroke	16
Gangrene and chronic infection	16
Hemorrhaging, severe	17
Paralysis (due to severe falls, electric shock, heart attacks and other unusual and dramatic traumas)	19
Poisonings	20
Rash and itching, acute (poison ivy, oak and sumach)	23
References	24

BASIC FIRST AID

Assuming more responsibility for your own body and the health problems it may encounter is becoming quite popular these days. "Self-health care is something we all espouse," said Dr. Allen Doumas, associate director of health of the American Medical Association's Department of Education. "It's a great way for people to take care of themselves."[1]

Recent statistics indicate that this trend is more widespread than many of us may realize. Consider this: Between 75 and 85 percent of all illnesses in Great Britain are now managed without doctor consultations.[2] Or how about the fact that nearly half of all *acute* conditions in the United States are now being treated without physician consultation?[3] In some cases, the percentage of symptoms treated without a visit to the doctor has been as high as 80 percent.[4]

But for the purposes of this booklet, our attention will mainly be devoted to yet another significant study, which found no difference in outcome between self-care and professional care for minor illnesses. According to this particular evaluation, individuals are just as capable of giving themselves the same kind and quality of adequate care for most minor problems as that provided by any medical doctor.[5] This speaks especially well for the relatively simple herbal treatments outlined in the present work and the value of assuming more responsibility for your own body.

A number of first aid situations—including those which qualify under the category of emergency medicine—and their respective methods and materials for treatment are given. Familiarity with them can undoubtedly save considerable expense in terms of medical costs.

Cuts, abrasions, minor wounds. Several popular American herbals have suggested capsicum or cayenne pepper (*Capsicum annuum*) to treat minor wounds. Powdered capsicum may be applied quite freely to open cuts and minor wounds in order to stop the bleeding.

But the seaweed kelp (*Laminaria* species) is far more efficacious in checking hemorrhages of this order. It makes a marvelous hemostatic agent because of the sodium alginate or alginic acid present in the herb. During World War II kelp was used extensively by the British to stop bleeding. A number of medical journals at the time carried articles about its value in this regard.[6]

Other powdered herbs that will work for this just as well are the following: yarrow (*Achillea millefolium*), wild geranium or cranesbill (*Geranium maculatum*), slippery elm (*Ulmus fulva*), goldenseal (*Hydrastis canadensis*), cinquefoil (*Potentilla canadensis*), and plantain (*Plantago lanceolata* and *P. major*).

Diarrhea. There are a great number of herbs that will help to correct a loose stool. Some herb books contain as many as a hundred and fifty plants useful in treating diarrhea.[7] For domestic use catnip (*Nepeta cataria*) and comfrey root are two that I recommend.

But the one which I prefer above all others is slippery elm bark. I have taken the powdered form of this bark with me wherever I have traveled in the world. In the Yucatan jungles of Mexico and in the faraway reaches of northern China, this herb has been a veritable lifesaver when I have suffered from acute cases of diarrhea. I have used both the bulk powder (about 2 teaspoons to 6 ounces of liquid) and capsules (6) to correct this embarrassing and annoying problem. Not only does the powdered bark tighten up a loose stool remarkably well, but it also strengthens the colon and the rest of the body with its many nutrients. A little cornstarch may sometimes be necessary in conjunction with the slippery elm if acute diarrhea fails to respond to the bark alone. Slippery elm is most compatible with pineapple juice, apple sauce or similar mild fruit products.

Frostbite. Administer a quarter cup of warm eucalyptus tea internally and rub the fingers, hands, toes and limbs with a lotion made of one part cayenne pepper and three parts brandy. Rub vigorously. Brandy may also be given internally. Or try some warm ginger tea to which a stick of cinnamon has been added for extra stimulating flavor.

Insect bites and stings, nonpoisonous. To reduce their pain, inflammation and itching, the following herbs may be used with success in the various forms recommended:

ALOE VERA *(Aloe vera)*—rub gel or salve on skin; apply poultice of liquid aloe vera.

CALENDULA OR MARIGOLD *(Calendula officinalis)*—rub salve, expressed juice from fresh plant or tincture on bite or sting.

COMFREY *(Symphytum officinale)*—rub on salve or apply a poultice of the freshly grated root or the powder (the allantoin in the root is responsible for the healing properties of the plant).

ELDER *(Sambucus* species, which includes *S. callicarpa* or Pacific red elderberry; *S. canadensis* or American elder; and *S. cerulea* or blueberry elder)—the leaves and flowers can be bruised, simmered down and the resulting lotion used to repel bees and other stinging insects or as a poultice for their stings and bites.[8]

GENTIAN *(Gentiana lutea)*—place freshly crushed leaves on afflicted areas. *Note:* Gentian is also a terrific blood builder when recuperating from a recent illness. It raises the white blood cell count in the body dramatically.

GOLDENROD *(Solidago virgaurea)*—apply a lotion made of the flowers to injured sites.

HOUND'S TONGUE *(Cynoglossum officinale)*—apply the bruised herb to insect bites.[9]

MUGWORT *(Artemisia vulgaris)*—bathe afflicted areas with strong decoction of either the herb or the rootstock.
FEVERFEW CHRYSANTHEMUM *(Chrysanthemum parthenium)* —rubbing the exposed parts of the body (hands, face, neck) with the flowers will keep bees, wasps and hornets away.
PENNYROYAL *(Mentha pulegium)*—rub some leaves on your hands, neck, arms or other exposed areas of the skin (or use the oil of pennyroyal instead) in order to repel mosquitoes, fleas and ticks.
WITCH HAZEL *(Hamamelis virginiana)*—use the lotion (available in any drugstore) as a good soothing agent for mosquito bites.

Other agents to use for bites and stings are an ice cube or an application of moistened Adolph's meat tenderizer upon the afflicted area (the papain from papaya fruit in the meat tenderizer is what works to give relief). However, one of the most effective remedies for the reduction of swellings due to insect bites and stings is to soak a wad of cotton with some Parson's or other household ammonia and then apply it to the afflicted area.

Nausea and dizziness. A tea made of any of the following herbs and taken when cool will relieve these conditions: chamomile *(Matricaria chamomilla)*; ginseng *(Panax* species) and Siberian ginseng *(Eleutherococcus)*; caraway seed *(Carum carvi)*; wild red raspberry *(Rubus strigosus)* and common raspberry *(R. idaeus)*. Capsules of either raspberry or Siberian ginseng may also be taken to alleviate nausea and dizziness due to travel sickness (i.e., airplane, ship, train or car).

Parasites. Those who travel to foreign countries where sanitary conditions may not be the best in the world would certainly do well to take some simple herbs along and to use them while staying in unsanitary environments. Ordinarily we would think of countries like Mexico and India as being examples of such places, but surprisingly even big nations that we regard as superpowers also fit this category. In 1979, when I went to the Soviet Union for several months, I found many parts of the USSR to be very unclean, to say the least. Leningrad was one of the worst places I've ever visited for unsanitary food and water. In fact, our Russian hosts warned us against drinking the water there, since it was highly contaminated with lead!

Herbs which I have taken with me to such places and have used with great success have been black walnut bark (*Juglans nigra*) and pumpkin seeds. They are best taken in capsulated form (about 4 to 6 per day of either one) for greater convenience.

Rash and itching. One of the simplest salve formulas for this is to take some goldenseal root powder (the amount depending on the area to be covered) and mix it with a little vitamin E oil (the best kind is from a veterinary supply house) until it has the smooth consistency of cooked cream of wheat cereal. Then add a little liquid honey and stir some more; this is to help the mixture adhere to the surface of the skin. Relief is obtained almost immediately after application to the afflicted area. Another effective salve is to stir equal parts of goldenseal and myrrh gum (*Commiphora myrrha*) into a base of oil (olive, safflower, sunflower) or grease (petroleum jelly, goose grease, bear fat).

Other herbs that may relieve these conditions may be found under Insect Bites and Stings.

Sunburn. Herbs recommended for mild sunburn and their methods of application are:

ALOE VERA—use the gel externally.

BURDOCK (*Arctium lappa*)—bathe the inflamed skin with a strong decoction of either the fresh leaves (preferred) or the root.

CHICKWEED (*Stellaria media*)—an ointment made of the freshly crushed leaves which have been mixed with lard or petroleum jelly will bring relief.

CUCUMBER (*Cucumis sativus*)—cucumber juice may be rubbed on the skin or a cucumber poultice may be applied.

  Note: Cucumber juice is also one of the very best things to dissolve uric acid accumulations in the form of gallstones and kidney stones. Good for chronic constipation, too.

PLANTAIN—lotion, salve or poultice made of fresh leaves and herb.

POPLAR OR QUAKING ASPEN *(Populus tremuloides)*—a tea made of either the bark or buds can be applied as a wash or a poultice; the buds boiled in olive oil or lard make an excellent salve.
PUMPKIN *(Cucurbita pepo)*—pumpkin seed oil is ideal for burns and chapped skin (either in summer or winter).
ST. JOHNSWORT *(Hypericum perforatum)*—an oil extract is good for burns.
WITCH HAZEL—the tincture provides soothing relief when applied and then fanned with a towel or electric fan for a few minutes.[10]

EMERGENCY MEDICINE

Bites and stings, poisonous (insects, snakes, scorpions, spiders, rabid animals, etc.). In the People's Republic of China (PRC), the very first thing that a barefoot doctor will do with a victim who has been bitten or stung by a poisonous creature is to *calm the patient;* this is done *before* tying a tourniquet, sucking out the poison, or doing anything else! This is an absolute prerequisite in order to keep the venom more localized.[11]

Herbs which would be of great value for calming the patient under such extreme conditions are asafetida *(Ferula fetida)*, German chamomile *(Matricaria chamomilla)*, or skullcap *(Scutellaria lateriflora)*. All three are antispasmodics and exert a powerful influence on the system to reduce any tension or excitement which might prevail during such an accident.

Doctors in China have a more forward-looking approach in the matter of poisonous bites and stings than we do in this country. The Chinese have formulated an interesting mixture of herbs indigenous to their part of the world which people can take in order to build up a lifelong immunity against such deadly venoms. This is worth evaluating here in terms of the lengthy protection it affords. In my transposition of these formulas, I am including some equivalent substitutes for a few of the ingredients used by the Chinese, since some of these plants are virtually impossible to find in our hemisphere. This unique kind of "herbal immunization" consists of the following materials and methods:

Parts	Chinese Name	Common Name	Latin Binomial
1.5 liang (1⅔ oz.)	pai-wei	white swallowwort (belonging to the milkweed family)	*Cynanchum vincetoxicum*

Note: An equal amount of pleurisy root (*Asclepias tuberosa*) may be substituted in place of this with similar results.

1.5 liang (1⅔ oz.)	pai-t'ou weng	nodding anemone	*Anemone cernua*
1.5 liang (1⅔ oz.)	hsu-chang-hsing		*Pycnostelma paniculatum*

Note: Two parts of pleurisy root and one part of ginger root (*Zingiber officinale*) may be substituted for the above two ingredients.

1 liang (1.1 oz.)	tu-hsing	a species of wild ginger	*Asarum blumei*

Note: Regular ginger root can be substituted in place of this. Ginger is successfully used in India for treating cobra bites and scorpion stings.[12]

1 liang (1.1 oz.)	pa-chiao-lien		*Dysosma auranticocaulis*

Note: Wild Oregon grape (*Mahonia aquifolium*) may be substituted in place of this.

1 liang (1.1 oz.)	lieh-hsieh chiu-hai-t'ang	split-leaf begonia	*Begonia lacinata*
5 ch'ien (½ oz.)	ch'ien-chin teng		*Stephania hernandifolia*

Note: American or Texas sarsaparilla or moonseed (*Menispermum canadense*) can be substituted. However, I recommend Spanish sarsaparilla (*Smilax officinalis*) for the novice, since the first sarsaparilla or moonseed is somewhat toxic and should only be used by experienced herbalists.

1 liang (1.1 oz.)	I-tien-hsueh		*Stephania* species

Note: Substitute an equal amount of Spanish sarsaparilla.

Prepare or obtain powders of all of the above ingredients. Mix together in the dry forms thoroughly. Combine approximately ½ oz. of the powder with a little bit of wine and take three times during the year (best during late spring or early winter), seven to ten days apart, at bedtime. For women and children, reduce the dosage. *Distilled* water can also be used in place of the wine to wash the powder down. Or mixture can be put into gelatin capsules; take 1 or 2 capsules three times a year, seven to ten days apart, at bedtime. *Not recommended* for children under twelve, pregnant women or women during their menstrual periods.

The Chinese guarantee that "if this regimen is faithfully followed, protection lasting one year against poisonous snakebites is acquired. This regimen, followed three years in a row (a combined total of nine doses), will confer lifelong protection against poisonous snakes and snake venom."[13]

For my own practical use, I have often relied upon equal parts of powdered ginger root, echinacea, red beet and skullcap in gelatin capsules (4 to 6 per day for three weeks of every quarter of the year) to provide me with some reasonable protection should I ever get bitten or stung by venomous creatures of any sort.

The Chinese barefoot doctors usually apply the standard tourniquets at least *twice* above the site of the injury or once on either side of the injury, spaced about two inches apart. Sometimes a third tourniquet is applied six or eight inches above the injury if necessary. The tourniquets or ropes used must be relaxed every thirty minutes for several seconds and the injured limb lowered, to prevent gangrene from setting in. After this, a small, clean knife should be used to open up the bite or sting itself. Pressure applied along the sides of the bite will force the venom out. At the same time, the bite should be washed with clear water. If no water is available, human urine may be used as a last resort, since it is usually highly antiseptic. The cupping technique should be used over the bite to draw out the poisoned blood. *A lit match or burning cigarette placed over the bite or sting can also be used to dissipate the toxic effect of the venom itself.* Only in extreme emergencies should the bite ever be sucked by mouth. And when this is required, the person doing the sucking should be very sure that there are no breaks or sores in the mucus membrane of the mouth and that the contents are spit out immediately and not retained for any length of time. A person with a lot of tooth fillings should not engage in such oral removal of the poison, as it will tend to accumulate in teeth and probably cause the jaw to swell to an enormous size. The mouth should repeatedly be rinsed with clear water after *each* sucking attempt.

Fresh cucumbers soaked in sulphur water for a week, dried for another week, and then crushed are also efficacious. The powder is placed around the affected area. A tobacco grease compress can also be applied over the affected area, or the area may be washed with a tobacco solution. *A strong solution of sagebrush or juniper berry teas taken internally will act as effective antidotes to such poisonings.* If the venom has reached the heart and the victim becomes comatose, give a *small* amount of arsenic disulfide (red arsenic or realgar powder used as pigment in painting and in fireworks for the blue fire) with several crushed garlic cloves in an appropriate amount of water.[14]

Elecampane (*Inula helenium*) or lobelia (*Lobelia inflata*) given on an empty stomach in tea form are two of the finest antidotes that I know of against rabies.

Australian scientists have invented a new product called Stigose, which brings almost instant relief to stings suffered from marine life (jellyfish, man-o-war), plants (stinging nettle) and stinging trees. The main ingredient is aluminum sulphate. Such aluminum salts may also be found in alum.[15]

Crushed yarrow, used fresh in a poultice and placed over any kind of spider bite will help to draw out venom that may have been implanted in the flesh.[16]

Blindness, temporary (caused by chemicals or acids). There are two quick and rather effective measures which can be applied for this. The first thing to do is to flood the eyes with cold water in order to wash away and maybe neutralize some of the offending irritants. Next, a tiny amount of cayenne pepper (*Capsicum annuum*) may be carefully placed in the eyes themselves. Only a *very small* amount should be used, since too much might further damage the injured organs. The capsicum is intended as a homeopathic agent, causing the eyes to produce an abundance of tears, for tears contain a number of healing factors which can begin to repair damaged optic nerves and other vital tissue if immediate treatment is commenced. Liquid solutions of clear aloe vera juice, ascorbic acid, or sucrose-dextrose are also helpful in restoring sight if the eyes are gently washed with them. Large amounts of vitamin C and about 50 mg of zinc should be taken internally if the eyes are temporarily damaged by chemicals of some sort.

Burns (first, second and third degree). The victim's burned parts should be immediately immersed in ice-cold water, crushed (shaved) ice or fresh snow, if available. When I burned my right arm severely a few years ago, I immediately ran outside and threw myself onto a bank of new snow; I lay there for about twenty minutes, covered with quilts, until the pain had subsided somewhat. In another instance, I threw a young friend of mine into a big cattle watering trough on our ranch out in the wilderness when part of his clothing accidentally caught fire.

If a large area of the body is burned, then it is necessary to administer some kind of special drink in order to keep the patient from going into shock. Two solutions are recommended for this: a) 0.3 g salt, .15 g sodium bicarbonate (baking soda), 0.005 g phenobarbital in 100 milliliters of water; b) strong, *cool* tea made of 3 parts skullcap, 2 parts valerian root, and 1 part hops.

The Chinese use a number of medicinal herbs for treating burns. For first and second degree burns over a small area of the body, equal parts of powdered goldthread (*Coptis* species) and great burnet (*Sanguisorba officinalis*) are lightly sprinkled over the damaged surfaces of the skin. Wild Oregon grape root or goldenseal root may also be substituted for goldthread, since all three of them contain the important constituent, berberine, which is valuable in treating burns.[17] Goldenrod (*Solidago odora*) may also hold considerable value when applied topically in lotion or powdered form.[18]

A solution for cleaning the burn, and wet compresses to be placed upon the same, is made in China by taking ½ oz. of knotweed (*Polygonum* species), 1½ oz. of honeysuckle (*Lonicera* species), and 1½ oz. of barberry (*Mahonia* or *Berberis* species) and simmering them in 6⅓ cups of water until the concoction is reduced to about 4½ cups. In China both honeysuckle and knotweed are used extensively as dusting agents and to wash burns.[19]

Hound's tongue (*Cynoglossum officinale*) has been used extensively for burns in the past, in wet compresses made from the tea.[20] In the sixteenth century, a French doctor named Ambroise Paré often employed the juice of fresh onions with great success in treating all kinds of burns. Other physicians who copied his method improved upon it by adding such things as poplar or quaking aspen (*Populus tremuloides*) leaves and plantain leaves to their expressed onion juice.[21] And during the Second World War certain Soviet scientists found that a paste prepared from a small amount of freshly macerated onion emitted volatile substances which killed within a few minutes any yeast, protozoa and bacteria that were exposed to them. They utilized this onion on a number of burns which their soldiers and citizenry suffered when the Germans invaded their country.[22]

Baking soda mixed with some olive oil and applied to the skin will not only help to heal a severe burn, but will also prevent any scarring if the area is adequately covered. I know this to be so from personal experience several years ago.

Tannic acid has also been used in many clinics and hospitals in the past for the treatment of surface burns. A number of reports in leading medical journals have shown the tremendous effectiveness which this has achieved. For the most part, wet compresses soaked with boric acid were supplied to the many victims treated.[23] A number of tree barks and leaves are especially high in tannic acid and would prove of great value in wet compresses that have been soaked in their teas and applied to burned skin. They are: sumac leaves (*Rhus glabra*); sweet gum leaves (*Liquidambar styraciflua*); bayberry or wax myrtle bark (*Myrica cerifera*); white oak bark (*Quercus alba*); blackberry leaves (*Rubus villosus*); magnolia bark (*Magnolia glauca*); sassafras (*Sassafras albidum*); the fruit of the unripe persimmon (*Diospyros virginiana*).[24] A more complete list of plants that have tannic acid may be found in certain popular herb books.[25]

Clay has been recommended for burns as well. According to one authority,

Burns treated with clay heal better and more rapidly and leave fewer scars than with other methods, especially if the clay is applied immediately.

Apply cold clay in thick poultices with gauze between the clay and the sore. After one hour remove the poultice. . . . Clay eliminates all risks of infection and absorbs all the impurities and foreign bodies apt to be found in the burn. It also eliminates the destroyed cells, enabling cellular rebuilding to occur. Renew the applications each day and night, changing them every hour until the appearance of new pink tissue is evidenced.

Acid-burns should be treated with clay; but alkaline ones with lemon-water instead.[26]

Zinc is a potent catalyst of wound healing. The ancient Egyptians used it topically in the form of calamine and since then zinc oxide, zinc sulfate and zinc stearates in the form of powders, salves and ointments have continued to be used. It is likely that some of the element is absorbed through the skin, particularly through injured and granulating tissues.[27] Zinc supplements from the health food store can be crushed up into a powder, mixed with a little olive oil or petroleum jelly and then applied topically to the burned flesh. Soon new tissue will appear and scarring will be reduced to a minimum.

The allantoin present in comfrey root is also of tremendous value in treating burns. British doctors in the past have utilized poultices made of the mashed root with great effectiveness. Comfrey allantoin is a great cell proliferant and builds new tissues in no time at all.[28]

The camphor in eucalyptus leaves and tea tree oil—both from Australia—are valuable in treating burns since they both keep infection from occurring.

The right kind of diet also plays an important role in the healing of burns. Medical research has shown that increasing the ratio of sulfur in the diet by the use of methionine increases the rate of healing. It is interesting that wound tissue that is going through a healing process contains larger amounts of sulfur than the same tissue when it has not been wounded.[29] Vegetables high in sulfur are those from the *Brassica* family—i.e., cabbage, kale, kohlrabi—garlic and watercress. Plants containing significant amounts of methionine are corn, soybean and comfrey. Thus wound healing can be dramatically increased by simply combining both groups of plants in the diet. Raw cabbage juice/watercress compresses would have additional value when used topically.

Vitamins A, D and C should not be overlooked either. Large doses taken internally during a severe burn will expedite the patient's recovery. Sometimes fish oil has even been applied to damaged skin with marvelous results.

During World War I pads of sphagnum moss were sterilized and saturated with water-diluted garlic juice and applied to burns suffered by many soldiers in Europe.[30]

Poultices of slippery elm bark or fenugreek seed (*Trigonella foenumgraecum*) are yet another proven remedy of great value when it comes to burned skin and flesh. A broth made of slippery elm bark may also be administered internally because of its many nutritional benefits to the system as a whole.

Choking. Get the victim to stand up, stand behind him or her, and pass your arms around the lower part of his or her ribs in a Russian bear hug. Clasp your wrists and give a sudden, forceful squeeze in the pit of the stomach. The air compressed in the chest will blow out the obstruction like a champagne cork. If the first attempt doesn't work, try the procedure again, only harder. This is known as the famous Heimlich maneuver, developed by my good friend, Dr. Henry Heimlich of Cincinnati, Ohio. This method has saved thousands of lives, although some agencies like the American Red Cross still prefer older but less reliable procedures. Slippery elm tea or papaya juice given immediately after the Heimlich maneuver will bring further relief to the victim. Any other mucilaginous herb such as fenugreek seed tea may be used as well.

Fevers (malaria, typhoid, spotted, etc.). There are certain herbs which the Chinese find efficacious for various kinds of fevers. For instance, magnolia bark, a species of wormwood (*Artemisia* species), a species of Solomon's seal (*Polygonatum officinale*), licorice root (*Glycyrrhiza glabra*) and fresh gypsum are all used in different concoctions (teas) for treating both malaria and typhoid. A species of skullcap (*Scutellaria baicalensis*) and several citrus rinds (dried tangerine and orange peels) also figure quite prominently in the list of herbs recommended for malaria, while a species of peony (*Paeonia albiflora*) is used extensively (along with other things) for typhoid.

In addition to these medicinal agents, the Chinese recommend certain nutritional items to help rebuild and supplement the body with those things it needs most for promoting good health. For example, consider the two simple preparations suggested for strengthening systems weakened by malaria.[31]

Concoction A

Part	Chinese Name	Common Name	Latin Binomial
1 liang (1.1 oz)	ho-shou-wu	species of knotweed	*Polygonum multiflorum*
3 ch'ien (⅓ oz)	chiang	fresh ginger	*Zingiber officinale*
10	—?—	large Chinese dates	*Zizyphus jujuba*

Concoction B

Part	Chinese Name	Common Name	Latin Binomial
5 ch'ien (½ oz)	tang-shen	species of bluebell	*Campanumaea pilosula*
5 ch'ien	kuei-chai kuei-pan	tortoise shell	

Note: Surprisingly rich in calcium, iodine, manganese, silicon, and iron.

Part	Chinese Name	Common Name	Latin Binomial
2 ch'ien (¼ oz)	wu-mei	black "prunes" Japanese apricots	*Prunus mume*

Several herbs which are ideal for combating raging fevers are those which have berberine in their rootstocks—i.e., goldenseal, wild Oregon grape, and yellow root (*Xanthorhiza simplicissima*). Berberine has been proven clinically to work well against malaria. It accomplishes this by exerting a profound influence on the spleen. Now the spleen is known to act as a filter to remove microorganisms such as bacteria and protozoa from the bloodstream. Malarial parasites occur in large quantities in this organ. Berberine will increase the volume of the spleen, thereby increasing its rhythmic contractions. In this way the malarial parasites are expelled into the bloodstream where they are later eliminated from the body in urination or fecal waste.[32] Any of these recommended herbs may be taken in capsule form.

But fevers should also be treated with herbs in *liquid* form. Herb teas that are good for this are chamomile, yarrow, boneset (*Eupatorium perfoliatum*), pleurisy root, and borage (*Borago officinalis*).[33] Myrrh and echinacea are also excellent, in capsulated form.

Vitamins A, D and C should be taken in large amounts during an attack of fever. Herbs that will nourish, strengthen and rebuild are slippery elm bark, fenugreek seed and flaxseed (*Linum unsitatissimum*). Mix equal parts of all three and serve in a broth or tea form.

Fractures and sprains. One of the very best plant materials for this is turmeric. Combined with a little hot water, the powdered herb is made into a paste which can be applied externally to the site of injury. This is then bandaged with a gauze dressing. Or the paste can be smeared on the gauze itself, which is wrapped around the injury. Turmeric is also good for contusions and bruises.[34]

Fresh mullein leaves are also ideal to use. They can be macerated and applied as a poultice. They are excellent for the reduction of swellings, particularly glandular enlargements (i.e., adenoids, lymph, etc.). Clay poultices are very useful, too, in the treatment and management of sprains and fractures.

In China splints made of willow, fir, thick cardboard or bamboo strippings are used most often to set fractures. A member of the thyme family and roots of clematis or Chinese bower (*Clematis chinensis*) are taken internally as a concoction to alleviate pain from external or internal injury and to promote better blood circulation. Honeysuckle and mugwort (*Artemisia vulgaris*) are used to bathe fractures, while a powdered or crushed mixture of violets, gotu kola (*Centella asiatica* or *hydrocotyl asiatica*), plantain, vervain and heal-all (*Prunella vulgaris*) are used to make a compress for them. During the final stages of fracture mending, a concoction of St. Johnswort, mulberry twigs (*Morus alba*) and wormwood are given to correct muscular atrophy.

Heat stroke. Any of the following herbs administered as *cool* teas will exert a mild, refrigerant effect upon the system: date leaves (any of the *Zizyphus* species will do); ginseng root (*Panax* species known as Korean ginseng); mulberry leaves; licorice root; peony rootbark; peppermint leaves (*Mentha piperita*).[35]

Gangrene and chronic infection. During World War II the British government treated many of their wounded with extracts of garlic. Some of these wounded were already in a gangrenous state, but garlic effectively eliminated the condition in all of those who were treated with it.[36] Other herbs that are extremely useful in the treatment of gangrene and may be used with great efficacy in either a powder (dust), wash (decoction) or poultice form are: yarrow, echinacea (very good), comfrey (root and leaves), chaparral, myrrh gum, poplar bark, white oak bark, goldenseal, smartweed or pleurisy root (the last three, combined in powdered form or in hot fomentations, are excellent).[37]

Take ¼ pound of powdered charcoal, one ounce of smartweed (*Polygonum punctatum*), put these into a pan and pour 1 pint of boiling water over them. Let steep twenty minutes. Then mix 2 tablespoons wholewheat flour and enough dry charcoal with this solution to make a poultice. Spread on a piece of gauze a little larger than the affected part, so that it will be well covered, apply, place another piece of gauze over it, and secure with a bandage. If the afflicted part is painful, add 1 tablespoonful of lobelia when steeping the herbs. You may use a little flaxseed meal or cornmeal to make the poultice stick together. When there is pus and ulceration, warm some hydrogen peroxide and bathe the affected part thoroughly, applying repeatedly and wiping off with a piece of cotton until the wound is absolutely clean. Do this before applying the poultice. Another excellent poultice is made of 2 tablespoons ground flaxseed (or flaxseed meal), 1 teaspoon goldenseal, and ½ teaspoon myrrh. Add enough hot water to make a paste. The paste must not be too stiff; it must be soft enough to penetrate. Apply as any other poultice. Renew every six hours, cleaning each time with peroxide if pus forms. Take the following internally: mix equal parts of skullcap, valerian, yellow dock (*Rumex crispus*) and buckthorn bark (*Rhamnus frangula*).

Use 1 heaping teaspoon to a cup of boiling water. Let steep for ½ hour. Take 1 cupful at least one hour before each meal and 1 cupful before going to bed at night.[38]

Hemorrhaging, severe. One of the best mixtures of herb powders to have around in case of extreme bleeding consists of the following: equal parts of powdered white oak bark (*Quercus alba*), yarrow and geranium; or just equal parts of the first two if geranium happens to be unavailable at the time. Half a part of either goldenseal root or myrrh gum in the powdered form may be substituted for geranium, but wherever possible geranium should be used for maximum effectiveness. This powdered mixture can be applied as a pressure compress over the injured site. Bleeding will usually stop within a minute or two.

Kelp and cayenne pepper may also be used as in minor cuts, but they are of limited value, I have found, when the blood is spurting out in great quantities. However, several popular American herbals have suggested cayenne for the treatment of less severe hemorrhaging and for bleeding ulcers.[39] In fact, one of America's largest multilevel herb companies, in Utah, originated after one of its owners used capsulated cayenne pepper to successfully treat his stomach ulcers nearly a decade ago.[40] Some medical doctors in this country have used cayenne with good advantage in controlling bleeding of the lungs or the womb.[41]

Kelp is more effective. I had occasion to use it recently in Michigan in an emergency situation, with excellent results. The injured party had had her face severely cut with glass in an automobile accident. After the woman had been carefully removed from the wrecked vehicle and placed on the ground on a blanket, I put a small scoop of kelp in my hands and began rubbing them together very lightly above her injured face. And wherever the kelp fell on her, the bleeding seemed to stop just moments afterward. I repeated this process until practically her entire face was covered with the green powder. And while it made the injury appear even more ghastly than it was—someone remarked that it looked as if gangrene had set in—it did check and effectively control the loss of any more blood until the paramedics arrived to take her to the local hospital for further treatment.

Another herb which works very well to stop excessive bleeding is *Urtica dioica*, better known as stinging nettle. Some herbalists have recommended it for this purpose.[42] And a few medical doctors in the past have conducted limited experiments to show that such recommendations are indeed based upon clinical facts. A Confederate surgeon by the name of Francis Porcher successfully stopped the bleeding of a sheep whose artery he had severed by applying lint covered with a sponge soaked in a cold infusion and then a decoction of stinging nettle. The doctor also observed that "the juice of the plant seemed to have some effect in coagulating fresh blood poured out into the hand." A patient of his who suffered from bloody urine was given a cold infusion made with 2 ounces of the plant in 1 pint of water, in doses of a full wineglass four times a day; this cleared up the condition in no time at all.[43] Great burnet (*Sanguisorba officinalis*) also coagulates blood quite well.[44]

In China, they use some interesting mixtures of their own devising with relative success to control hemorrhaging. Here are several examples:

1. Equal parts of the following ingredients are first pulverized, then roasted in an oven until yellowish-black, and finally put over the point of bleeding as a compress:

Chinese Name	Common Name	Latin Binomial
t'ien-pien chu	aster	*Aster trinervius*
wu-pao hsieh	blackberry (leaves)	*Rubus tephordes*
t'ung-hao, huo-pa-kuo	pyracantha (berries)	*Pyracantha fortuneana*
p'u-huang	common cattail	*Typha latifolia*

2. Another mixture calls for the following:

Parts	Chinese Name	Common Name	Latin Binomial
4	tzu-chu ts'ao	Beautyberry sourbush French mulberry	*Callicarpa pedunculata* *C. Americana* (American species)
3	kang-nien	downy rosemyrtle	*Rhodomyrtus tomentosa*
3	san-ya	prickly ash	*Evodia lepta* or *Zanthoxylum roxburghianum*

3. Here is a third mixture of equal importance:

Parts	Chinese Name	Common Name	Latin Binomial
1 liang (1.1 oz.)	chiang t'an	ashes of ginger root	Zingiber officinale
1 liang	wu-ming-I	powdered manganese supplement	
1 liang	pai-chi	a plant of the orchid family somewhat related to a lady's slipper (Cypripedium pubescens)	Bletilla striata
5 chi'ien (½ oz.)	chi-nei-chin	unidentifiable (catnip comes closest to the properties of this herb)	unidentifiable
1 ch'ien (.11 oz.)		rock sugar	

This mixture is stored in airtight bottles and used for sprinkling over wounds and points of bleeding prior to bandaging.

The burned ashes of p'u-huang or common cattail are stored in a bottle once they've cooled and are used when needed. They are sprinkled liberally upon any external sites of profuse bleeding. They check extreme hemorrhaging remarkably well.[45]

Paralysis (due to severe falls, electric shock, heart attacks and other unusual and dramatic traumas).

In the People's Republic of China at least three different approaches are considered together in treating such a nervous and muscular disorder. First of all, certain herbs are used to stimulate blood circulation and provide badly needed energy to those parts most severely afflicted. A concoction of licorice root, ginger root and ordinary cinnamon sticks is used most often. Then the Chinese practice either acupuncture, acupressure (known in America as reflexology), various kinds of massage or a combination of all three on the patient. The rolling technique is a back-and-forth motion practiced on the spinal column from the cervical vertebrae to the fifth thoracic vertebrae for five to ten minutes, using light gentle motions. A vigorous rubbing technique is also employed, most generally on the arms and legs until such limbs become warm. Olive oil is sometimes used as a lubricant for this. The grasping technique is still another form of massage applied to the arms and leg calves down to the ankles.[46]

Jethro Kloss also successfully treated paralysis with herbs and massage. First he would give the paralyzed victim an enema. This would be followed by hot and cold applications to the spine, stomach and liver. After this would come hot and cold towel rubs, followed by a thorough massage over the entire body from head to foot. In cases of complete paralysis this entire process would be repeated many times and kept up for hours on end until some marked improvement was noticed, at which time the same routine would be continued but at a much reduced pace. According to him, he was able to cure even the most difficult types of paralysis if caught in the beginning stages and patiently worked with over an extended period of time.[47]

Poisonings.

FOOD POISONING. Burdock root tea is good for neutralizing certain poisons and for eliminating them from the system as well.[48] Horehound tea is an excellent antidote for all types of seafood poisoning, especially those resulting from the consumption of crab and lobster. Horehound (*Marrubium vulgare*) is also useful in other types of food poisoning—E. coli, salmonella, and the like.[49] A cooked concoction of mung beans and licorice root is also good to use.[50]

DRUG OVERDOSE AND ADDICTION. Various detoxification brews have been formulated by persons working with drug addicts. One such brew calls for equal parts of comfrey, mullein and spearmint, with smaller amounts of rose hips and orange peel, and just a pinch of goldenseal added when the tea is ready to drink. Not only does it help to clean out the opiates in the body, but it also helps to kick the habit.[51] A good liquid chlorophyll or green drink (8 oz. glass) at least three times a day is also valuable. This detox brew was taken by one addict going through the withdrawal symptoms from heroin and was found to be of particular benefit.[52]

The detox brew will work for those who have been addicted to alcohol, heroin, methadone, cocaine, tranquilizers, amphetamines, marijuana, PCP (angel dust), LSD, caffeine and tobacco. And in many cases, when withdrawal stress becomes too unbearable, a special relaxant brew may be of tremendous help. Such a "relaxo brew" consists of equal portions of spearmint, chamomile and valerian root.[53]

Vitamins are also essential for the treatment of drug addiction. If some vitamin E oil is rubbed on the "tracks" of prolonged self-injection of drugs twice a day, the healing of the scars begins to be noticed within four days as a general rule.[54] Vitamin C also has a profound detoxicating effect on those who have smoked marijuana, especially that which originates in Mexico and has usually been sprayed with the poisonous chemical paraquat. Megadoses of C are recommended in such cases for maximum results.[55]

Activated charcoal, glucagon and doxapram are often used on OD cases that have advanced to a comatose state.[56] One-third part eucalyptus and two-thirds parts of horehound tea, slightly warm, may also be judiciously administered to overcome such comas.

Recently scientists have formulated a unique combination of fourteen well-identified species of higher plants, whose extracts were obtained through an enzymatic process with macroenzymes in the laboratory. The combination is called "neoalleviase (NA-1700)" and has shown extremely promising results in the suppression of withdrawal signs and symptoms of heroin addicts.[57]

RADIATION. The seaweed kelp can absorb a lot of radiation from fluid materials and from within the body itself. Its use is highly recommended for this problem.[58] Other seaweeds such as dulse, Irish moss, Iceland moss and assorted algaes also work in the same way as kelp. Clay is another good adsorbent for radioactive isotopes within the body. So is St. Johnswort, garlic and aloe vera. In fact, if a little (4 oz.) liquid aloe vera is consumed each morning, it will help to heal tissue that may have been damaged by cobalt or X-ray radiation. Slippery elm and fenugreek are also wonderful mucilages to take for excess radiation.

HOUSEHOLD CLEANING AGENTS *(lye, toilet bowl cleaner, etc.).* Milk or water will help to neutralize these agents. Olive oil, fenugreek seed or slippery elm teas will help to ease the pain.

FUMES *(kerosene, carbon monoxide, gas, etc.).* Raw radish juice in small quantities, liquid fructose, raw beet juice laced with a little cayenne pepper or strong, black coffee are all good to use *separately* once the victim has regained some consciousness and is able to take any one of them internally.[59]

PLANTS *(toadstools, harmful berries and beans, etc.).* Activated charcoal is highly recommended for these types of poisonings. White oak bark, orange pekoe, black, oolong or some other herbal teas that are high in tannic acid may also be employed with good success. A magnesium supplement should be administered along with any of the above.[60] More important, herbs such as dandelion root or peach bark in tea form *and a high protein diet* are invaluable to use in mushroom poisoning in order to prevent severe damage to the liver.[61]

HEAVY METALS *(lead, cadmium, mercury, etc.).* Burdock root tea, wild Oregon grape root tea, powdered goldenseal root (capsule form) and, surprisingly, even some blue cheeses like gorgonzola are some good remedies in cases of lead poisoning. The cheese mold is especially good as an oral chelating agent for the lead. Garlic and onion are also very good for lead and cadmium alike, especially in cases of slow accumulation over a lengthy period of time. A powdered protein drink or foods such as milk or eggs are used to inactivate the mercury located within the body. Both clay and seaweeds might also have some limited value, depending, of course, on the severity of the poisoning.[62]

INSECTICIDES *(DDT and related herbicides).* Kelp and other herbs high in sodium should be taken. A low fat, high carbohydrate, high protein diet is recommended to avoid liver or kidney damage. A concoction of tangkuei or dongguei (Chinese angelica), rhubarb root, licorice root and a little white alum are to be taken internally as a purgative.[63]

For arsenic poisoning, either large amounts of burdock root tea, strong black coffee, or plain sagebrush tea are all excellent remedies.

Acute rash and itching (poison ivy, oak and sumach). See under *Basic First Aid* the entries for "Rash and Itching." Jewelweed (*Impatiens pallida, I. capensis* and *I. biflora*) is a very effective antidote against poison ivy and its relatives. In the early 1950s the USDA confirmed the old wives' tale about jewelweed being good for skin eruptions when it discovered a certain fungicide principle in the plant that was excellent for treating athlete's foot and certain types of dermatitis. Since then several commercial lotions now on the market contain extracts of this herb under the listing of 2-methoxy-1, 4-naphthoquinone among the ingredients. Some of the fresh juice can be smeared on the skin if an itch commences. Or the sap can be made into a soothing lotion for use on irritated skin. Cover a panful of the herb with water and boil the liquid down to *half* of its original volume. The strained juice can then be directly applied to prevent an outbreak from occurring. Or it can be frozen in ice cube trays for later use. Once the squares have solidified, transfer the medicated ice to a plastic bag and store it in the freezer. Thus, if you should find yourself nursing a bad bout of itching in a season when jewelweed is unavailable, simply melt some of the frozen juice, smearing it generously over the infected area.[64]

Using aloe vera gel and increasing vitamin C intake to 5,000 milligrams per day will afford relief as well.[65] Fantastic relief from the itching can also be obtained by letting tap water run intermittently over the afflicted area (ideal for hives and shingles too). Or how about soaking such parts in a strong cool solution of peppermint tea (the menthol affords great relief) or cool mugwort tea? It is the urushiol in these plants (poison ivy, oak, and sumac) which causes the dermatitis.[66]

REFERENCES

1. *Republic Scene.* October 1981, p. 62.
2. Dunnell, K., and Cartwright, A. 1972. *Medicine Takers. Prescribers and Hoarders.* London: Routledge & Kegan Paul.; *Journal of the Royal College of General Practitioners.* 1973. 23:255–66; *Royal Society Health Journal.* 1977, 97:159–64.
3. *Acute Condition Incidence and Associated Disability.* 1977. Washington, D.C.: U.S. Department of Health, Education and Welfare, Publication No. PHS 78-1553.
4. *New England Journal of Medicine.* 1979, 300:535–37.
5. *Journal of the Royal College of General Practitioners.* 1977, 27:155–59.
6. *British Journal of Surgery.* January 1950, 37:307; *Annals of Surgery.* January 1947, 125:102; 113–14; *Lancet.* October 28, 1948, p. 651; *Quarterly Journal of Experimental Physiology.* 1947, 31:26, 28–29.
7. Lust, John. 1979. *The Herb Book.* New York: Bantam Books, p. 66.
8. Fielder, Mildred. 1982. *Fielder's Herbal Helper for Hunters, Trappers, and Fishermen.* Tulsa: Winchester Press, pp. 3–13.
9. Lust. *The Herb Book,* pp. 92, 143, 162, 208–209, 234, 412–13.
10. Lust. *The Herb Book,* pp. 140, 155, 168, 318, 324, 344.
11. *The Official Chinese Paramedical Manual;* publ. in the U.S. as *A Barefoot Doctor's Manual.* 1977. Seattle: Cloudburst Press.
12. Chopra, Col. Sir R. N. 1958. *Chopra's Indigenous Drugs of India.* Calcutta: U.N. Dhur & Sons Private Ltd., pp. 608, 610.
13. *A Barefoot Doctor's Manual,* p. 73.
14. *A Barefoot Doctor's Manual,* p. 75.
15. *Medical Journal of Australia.* August 9, 1980, pp. 146–50.
16. Fielder. *Fielder's Herbal Helper,* p. 3.
17. *A Barefoot Doctor's Manual,* p. 70; Culbreth, David M. R., M.D. *A Manual of Materia Medica and Pharmacology.* Philadelphia. p. 199.
18. Lust. *The Herb Book,* pp. 208–209.
19. *A Barefoot Doctor's Manual,* p. 70.
20. Lust. *The Herb Book,* pp. 234–35.
21. *Bulletin of the History of Medicine.* February 1944, 15:145, 147.

22. *American Review of Soviet Medicine.* February 1944, I:236–50.
23. *Surgery, Gynecology, and Obstetrics.* 1925, 41:202–21; *Annals of Surgery.* July 1926, 84:19–36; *Archives of Surgery.* 1929, 18:803–806.
24. Porcher, Francis Peyre. 1863. *Resources of the Southern Fields and Forests.* Charleston: pp. 344–47.
25. Lust. *The Herb Book,* p. 51 (under astringents).
26. *Well-Being.* 29:12.
27. *Annals of Surgery.* 1967, 165:432.
28. Hills, Lawrence D. 1976. *Comfrey—Fodder, Food and Remedy.* New York: Universe Books, pp. 200–203.
29. *Proceedings of the Society for Experimental Biology and Medicine.* 1957, 77:305.
30. Hylton, William H. 1978. *The Rodale Herb Book.* Emmaus, PA: Rodale Press, p. 449.
31. *A Barefoot Doctor's Manual,* pp. 107–111.
32. Chopra. *Chopra's Indigenous Drugs of India,* pp. 294–95.
33. Kloss, Jethro. 1939. *Back to Eden.* Santa Barbara, CA: Woodbridge Press, 1981 edition, pp. 349, 425–426.
34. *CRC Critical Reviews in Food Science and Nutrition.* 1980. 12:291, no. 3.
35. *A Barefoot Doctor's Manual,* pp. 175–176.
36. Adams, Rex. 1977. *Miracle Medicine Foods.* West Nyack, NY: Parker Publishing Co., p. 18.
37. Kloss. *Back to Eden,* p. 350.
38. Kloss. *Back to Eden,* pp. 431–32.
39. Christopher, John R. 1976. *School of Natural Healing.* Provo, Utah: Bi-World Publishers, p. 407; Kloss. *Back to Eden,* p. 216.
40. Brailsford, Kenneth E. 1979. *How I Made a Million Dollars in the Herb Business.* Provo, Utah: Bi-World Publishers.
41. Shoemaker, John V., M.D. 1908. *A Practical Treatise on Materia Medica and Therapeutics.* Philadelphia: F. A. Davis Co., p. 314.
42. Lust. *The Herb Book,* p. 291.
43. Porcher. *Resources of the Southern Fields and Forests,* pp. 269–70.
44. Lust. *The Herb Book,* p. 212.
45. *A Barefoot Doctor's Manual,* p. 64.
46. *A Barefoot Doctor's Manual,* p. 103.
47. Kloss. *Back to Eden,* pp. 17–18.
48. Lust. *The Herb Book,* p. 140.
49. *A Barefoot Doctor's Manual,* p. 313.
50. *A Barefoot Doctor's Manual,* p. 76.

51. *Well-Being*, 28:11.
52. *Well-Being*, 40:63.
53. *Vegetarian Times/Well-Being*. 42:62.
54. *Vegetarian Times*. January-February 1979, p. 45.
55. *General Pharmacology*. 1980, 11:455–61.
56. *Clinical Toxicology*. 1980, 16:395–96.
57. *International Journal of Addictions*. 1980, 15:883–87.
58. *Sewage Industrial Wastes*. 1959, 31:1409–15; *Radiation Botany*. 1974, 14:37; Airola, Paavo. 1976. *How To Get Well*. Phoenix, AZ: Health Plus Publishers, pp. 173–74.
59. *A Barefoot Doctor's Manual*, p. 75.
60. *American Family Physician*. November 1979, pp. 155–56.
61. *Clinical Symposia*. 1978, 30(2):30.
62. *Clinical Symposia*, pp. 31–32.
63. *Clinical Symposia*, p. 33; *A Barefoot Doctor's Manual*, p. 76.
64. *Bestways*. August 1978, p. 77; *Mother Earth News*. March-April 1981, 68:8.
65. *Total Health*. August 1980, p. 38.
66. *Journal of Pharmaceutical Sciences*. May 1980, 69:588–89.
67. *A Barefoot Doctor's Manual*, p. 72.